The Gift of Courage

The Gift of Courage

James Wilkes

Second Edition
Revised and Enlarged

The Anglican Book Centre
Toronto, Canada

To Elizabeth,
my wife

Contents

Introduction

From the time that I first remember thinking seriously about the teachings of the church, I had trouble accepting what seemed to be magic elements in what was being taught. Early in school we learned that water, because of the pull of gravity, seeks its own level. How, then, did the Red Sea divide? And can sticks become serpents? And can a bush really burn without being consumed? I wondered how Jesus could have walked on water. But I was loyal to the group, and if I had to believe these things in order to stay with them, then believe them I would!

The problem didn't get any easier when I entered medical school. As my scientific knowledge of physiology and disease grew, the acceptance of Jesus' healing miracles became more difficult. The raising of Lazarus, after Martha had warned that his body would smell from decomposition, was terribly hard to accept. I found myself becoming irritated, and worried that God might be capricious. Why just Lazarus, the widow's son, and the little girl? Why not more? Why just then? Why not now? Even more disturbing was the thought that if God was capricious, how could he be trusted? I had to consciously put these ideas aside, saying to myself that, after all, the miracles weren't so important to the faith, and there were many mysteries that we couldn't comprehend.

I lived in the shelter of that cocoon until I entered seminary. It was there that I was exposed to biblical criticism and discovered that these problematical stories need to be seen in a theological context that lies beyond factual history. These special and important stories deepen our understanding of God's action in history, and of life itself. No longer did I have to place my scientific knowledge in limbo. I was free to question and appraise without doing violence to the truth as I saw it.

The experience was at once exciting and terrifying! God's action in history takes place through men and women, or in Paul's phrase, he puts his spirit in earthen vessels. The actual Scriptures themselves were written by human beings—people gifted by special grace, no doubt, but human nevertheless—who thought, puzzled, and made choices to include certain ideas and images and to exclude others. This whole way of thinking deepened my understanding of history itself. I saw history as not just a collection and explanation of facts but the unfolding of reality. The day-to-day lives of men and women were not simply the putting in of time but the very stuff of God's action. From this perspective the whole of life possesses a religious significance.

It is disappointing that men and women of science have often been asked to speak for the church in a fashion that tends to perpetuate a kind of dualism. On the one hand there is the faith and spiritual salvation, and on the other hand, the material world. These two may coexist, and sometimes harmoniously, but there is no apparent relationship between them. The nuclear physicist may rhapsodize over the structures and forces in matter, and even proclaim that his or her belief in God stemmed from appreciation of these wonders. In the same fashion the physician may express admiration for the complexities of God's creation in the organization of the human body.

After the scientists have spoken, we may be left with a sense of pleasure, or even confidence, that an appreciation of creation can lead to a deepening of one's religious belief. However, we are often left with a sense of God being "out there" and "back then," and his created order existing here and now. One cannot quarrel with such statements from the scientists, but too many statements of this kind tend to obscure the more important point—that matter exists, and human bodies exist, in order that history can be made now or, put another way, in order that people can do things. Creation is still going on. It is this simple message that is so profoundly religious.

The importance of each person's history was impressed further on me through my studies in psychiatry. The psychotherapist knows the importance of helping a person to accept his or her own history and to come to terms with the things that he or she has done. The therapist is also acquainted with the hazards and pitfalls of making plans on the basis of wishful thinking rather than on an accurate assessment of facts and experience, or of building personal relationships on what is wanted from another rather than on what is possible from another. The health of a person depends on his or her success in struggling through all the illusions of life, which are so beguiling, into the realities of life, which at times seem so stern and forbidding.

Therapists, in their sensitivity and compassion, need not be harsh in attempting to show up illusion for what it is. At times the fight can become unbearable, and pausing in the distraction and apparent peacefulness of illusion may give a person a chance to rest and catch his or her breath. But the road to health and growth requires the eventual shedding of each sheltering illusion and the moving forward into reality.

This journey through the clouds of illusion into the light of reality cannot be done on effort alone, nor can it be done with exhortation or explanation, as helpful as all these things may be. The movement forward through illusion into reality cannot be accomplished without one of God's special gifts —*the gift of courage.*

Thoughts on these matters would come to my mind as I continued in the practice of psychiatry.

It was then that I was fortunate enough to meet the Rev. Colin Proudman, principal of the College of Emmanuel and St. Chad, the Anglican Theological Seminary at the University of Saskatchewan. He encouraged me to put my thoughts in writing so that I could give the four lectures that comprise the Martin Lectures, the annual lectureship at his college. I will always be grateful to him for giving me the impetus to think more fully on these matters.

Except for some minor changes, Chapters 1 through 4 of this book are as they were spoken. They were initially addressed to what was primarily, although not exclusively, an audience of clergy. Chapter 5, an article, originally published in *Re:Action,* Spring 1980, by the Metropolitan Toronto Branch of the Canadian Mental Health Association, is used here by permission; it has been reworked for this publication. It is added to this book to give a secular balance to the material. While suggestions of the themes and ideas in the first four chapters may appear in the fifth, the new context may help the reader to a further understanding.

In the process of working through this material, I became struck by the truth that as magic and illusion are lifted from life, the mystery deepens. At first this idea seemed paradoxical to me, but on reflection it is not. Magic and illusion disguise and hide reality—they are the opposite of mystery; they are banal. Mystery is found in the action of God in the lives and history of men and women.

I would like to thank James Reed, David Clark, Paul Gibson, and Donald Anderson, my friends and priests of the church, whose support and criticisms were essential to this book; and Erma Gerry, who so willingly typed and retyped the numerous drafts.

J.W.

1.
The Reality of Evil

The mind and the soul are two great and essential attributes of human nature. Both have fascinated, bemused, and intrigued humankind through the ages. Both will figure largely in the substance of this book. Human attitudes and understandings continue to shift, and as they do, the meaning of words shifts with them. This is no less true for the meanings of "mind" and "soul." The Greek words for "mind" and "soul" are *nous* and *psyche*. Modern sensibilities might be somewhat shattered to think that the word "psychology" really refers to the science or study of the soul. Perhaps today the word "nousology" would more closely reflect the subject matter of those who profess to study the mind. But despite their ever-changing meaning, these two words have always provided a means for the exploration and understanding of the human condition.

Psychiatry and religion might be likened to two great ships of discovery. These ships chart their separate voyages to suit their own purposes, they develop language, instruments, and tools befitting their particular experience, and those aboard, like those serving in all great ships, develop a loyalty to one another and to the ship in which they sail. In the climate of today the meeting of these two ships can provide either an opportunity for the mutual exchange of information and technique or the possibility of a dockside brawl. On the one hand, nourished by respect and admiration, there is open cooperation and sharing; and on the other hand, fueled by mistrust and jealousy, there is isolation and condemnation. This book tries to take advantage of the constructive opportunities. The argument is based on the premise that a person's health and wholeness are best served by mind and body being in harmony, and psychiatry and religion being in a state of concord. The argument also affirms that psychiatry requires a soul while religion requires actual human experience.

It is hoped that these discussions will by argument and illustration support the position that the ability to understand human beings and their behavior, and therefore the capacity to help and strengthen them, can be enhanced and sustained by basing such understanding on religious principles. For therapists and clinicians this does not mean that they must relinquish their dynamic understanding and their transactional skills, but that they should allow such understanding and skills to be informed by religion. These discussions deal with ways in which religion might serve to inform those who are engaged in the work of healing troubled people.

The religious position in these discussions is taken from the Judeo-Christian tradition. It is the tradition in which the writer was raised. The absence of other religious positions is to be taken not as a bias for exclusivity, but as a recognition of unfamiliarity and ignorance.

The mutual exchange and nourishment between workers in mental health and workers in religious and pastoral pursuits have already been of great benefit to humankind and have deepened people's understanding of themselves. There continues to be a prodigious amount of material written and spoken in what might be called the dialogue between psychiatry and religion.[1]

One can go into church or synagogue today and hear sermons with psychological and sociological content that might well fit into a program of in-service education for the staff of a mental health clinic. One can ask someone for mental relief and be given advice that might be questioned in the light of traditional Christian moral principles. Will there be a dockside brawl or mutual sharing and enlightenment? The difficulty in such meetings has been, and will continue to be, finding a common language and holding to a common purpose.

It seems that a useful common starting point for those who travel in either ship is *people in difficulty, trouble, or perplexity.* There appears to be some sort of naiveté, simplicity, or perhaps egocentricity in people that leads them to start questioning their reality and the meaning of things, especially when things are not going well for them. They may reflect on reality on other occasions, but times of pain seem to have a particular capacity to arouse questioning and reflection.

There appear to be two contrasting responses to pain and brokenness: one is to confront, question, and reflect on them; the other is to deny them and try to escape from them. It is the fear of this pain (the pain which is part of the human condition) that gives root to much of the destruction and imprisonment in the lives of men and women today.

For the purpose of this discussion, we shall think of two kinds of pain. The first is physiological pain that comes from excitation of the body's pain fibers because of disease or trauma. This pain can, by appropriate therapeutic intervention, be largely controlled. The second kind of pain is central to this discussion and is that which comes from humankind's existential alienation. This pain is part of the human condition and cannot be taken away. It has to be faced and not avoided!

In this attempt to avoid pain, people have devised escape techniques that, because of human ingenuity, are numberless. They have endorsed the notion that the avoidance of pain is an end in itself and have set up pleasure spas. They have picked on the word "therapeutic" and regarded as therapeutic anything that makes one feel good or permits one to do one's own thing. Such solutions never ask whether feeling good is the result of being destructive or cruel to others. Indeed, the trick becomes for those pursuers of pleasure to attack any world view that seeks the meaning of human existence. They develop a language that talks of commitment as a "heavy," of permanence as boring—a language that talks of sexuality in terms of technique and lacks the roots to understand sexual experience expressed in the Bible as "knowing." Some find a defense against pain in the illusion that an experience of self-discovery has made them "free." They have wondrously screamed their pain away or have found that they need not burden themselves with the pain of others. They are told they need only "relate" if they should happen to meet. In the fear of the forces arising from the unconscious, people have imprisoned themselves in rigid thought patterns and heavy technology which, unless nourished by some life-giving force, threatens to erase life from this planet.

The attempt to escape or deny pain will eventually bring on more pain; the answer lies not in turning away from it but in meeting it. This is not an argument for masochism, but somehow we must grapple with pain, struggle with it, confront it, and try to understand it. We must not avoid pain or flee from it; we must diagnose it, name the demons, and begin to dispel their destructive powers. The naming of demons is not magic but the conscious acknowledgment and identification of the destructive powers around us. It is when we cannot see our opponent that we are vulnerable and more easily confused. The devil, we are told, is like a roaring lion who prowls around looking for someone to devour. He puts on many disguises, but it is important that we name him, and continue to name and rename him, however endless and arduous the task may be. We will look more fully at pain and suffering in a later chapter, but for the moment the main point is this: that in turning away from the pain in life people are in danger of losing themselves. They need help in maintaining an accurate reading on the reality which includes pain.

In the language at the dockside there is a word that can help keep people on course. It is a word seldom used by those traveling in the ship of the mind, but commonly seen and feared by those traveling in the ship of the soul. The word is "evil," a word with deep moral and religious significance. Evil is an essential reality of human experience. It should in no way be confused with magic or be related to some occult or mysterious influence. Evil is real; it is part of life. The prison that people find themselves in, when they are beset by anxiety and unable to function in their work, may be called neurotic from a psychological sense, but it is also evil. The incapacity of a person to form trusting relationships, when he or she brings a marriage to an end and leaves the children unsure, guilty, and disconsolate, may be called immaturity, but it is evil. This immaturity may in large part be explained by the dynamic transactions and experiences of his or her life, but even so, there is no escape from the evil facts. Any notion of evil as being funny or connected to a little figure with a pointed tail is dispelled by reading the morning paper or looking into the anguished faces of those who experience the cruelty and vindictiveness of their fellow human beings. Evil is not funny; it is real. If we are to be healthy, we must take it seriously, and we must confront and deal with it or fall into confusion, apathy, and decay.

Evil, in the way we are talking about it here, is not simply the absence of good. The Swiss psychiatrist C. G. Jung has written: "There is no getting round the fact that if you allow substantiality to good, you must also allow it to evil. If evil has no substance, good must remain shadowy, for there is no substantial opponent for it to defend itself against, but only a shadow, a mere privation of good. Such a view can hardly be squared with observed reality."[2] Evil has a reality of its own which permeates the physical and spiritual dimensions of our existence. One is reminded of Solzhenitsyn's words from *The Gulag Archipelago:* "The line separating good and evil passes not through states, nor between classes, nor between political parties either—but right through every human heart."[3]

Paul Ricoeur, in his book *The Symbolism of Evil,*[4] attempts an analysis of evil. He writes that evil is not nothing, and not even something external to human beings, but something intrinsic to their very existence. Ricoeur helps us understand evil as that which disorients people from what is real. He illustrates with the Adamic myth from Genesis. When God's commandment not to eat the fruit of the tree becomes opposed to Adam's own will—his "other" rather than his "orient"—the function of the commandment changes, and Adam is vulnerable. Instead of seeing God's law as a boundary for his existence and a support for his reality, he regards it as an imposition and turns away from it. Evil takes root at the point of the individual's disorientation from the larger reality.

Ricoeur goes on to remind us that the word "evil" is a symbol and that the world of symbols is not tranquil. Every symbol is iconoclastic in comparison to some other symbols and tends to defend itself with accumulated meanings, to thicken and solidify into what Ricoeur calls an "idolatry." The symbol must be open to newness of image and understanding. Our idea of evil will continue to change and develop, but this should not prevent us from continuing to use the same word to help us understand more clearly the world around us.

This religious word "evil" assists the mental health worker not when it appeals to magic or mysterious power plays, not when it leads to an attempt to avoid the hard work and struggle of therapy, and not when it seeks to avoid the risk and commitment necessary for the molding of healing relationships. This religious word "evil" is of help precisely when it identifies hurt, confusion, and brokenness as significant. When the word "evil" is applied to the brokenness of human life, it demands that we take seriously the pain of our brother or sister before us. It demands that we not laugh at it or make light of it. It demands that we use our diagnostic terms and categories to clarify our therapeutic plans and not to explain the total reality of a person's predicament. Religion does not tell mental health workers to stop what they are doing and to start praying; rather it encourages them to a more proficient and compassionate use of the skills they already have.

When the term "evil" is applied to the list of psychiatric diagnoses, to the various psychological or sociological formulations for the destructive and dehumanizing events of human life, or to the geographic and biological explanations of the world's ecological problems, then one is saying that such realities are of eternal consequence. The application of this religious term to these scientific ideas gives depth to both disciplines—religion is grounded in experience, and science is nourished with a soul—and each helps the other from falling into idolatry.

The recognition of evil, we are arguing, is important in maintaining humankind's orientation to reality. We need ways of recognizing and understanding evil so that we may be better able to deal with it. Paul Tillich provides us with a useful tool for recognizing evil in his discussion of existential anxiety.[5] Existential anxiety is not to be confused with the word "anxiety" as it is used in referring to feelings of tenseness, or with the way the word is used by the psychoanalyst. Tillich begins his discussion of existential anxiety by talking about the reality of being and of nonbeing. In simple terms nonbeing is the background for being—that into which all existence is set. For this reason, Tillich sees nonbeing as a condition or part of reality, and he points to the importance in human life of affirming one's self, not by denying nonbeing, but in spite of the threat of nonbeing. It is the threat that nonbeing imposes on one's self-affirmation that gives rise to existential anxiety. However, because existential anxiety is essential to the human condition, it is necessary to take this anxiety upon oneself. For the purpose of this discussion, we would add that avoiding the burden of existential anxiety is evil and can be shown to underlie much of the brokenness and alienation in human life.

According to Tillich, one's self-affirmation can be seen in three modes. The first mode he calls ontic self-affirmation, which, in simple terms, would include one's historical presence and action —the events in a life. Nonbeing threatens one's ontic self-affirmation *relatively* in terms of fate, and *absolutely* in terms of death. The second mode he calls spiritual self-affirmation—the meaning in a life—and nonbeing threatens one's spiritual self-affirmation *relatively* in terms of emptiness, and *absolutely* in terms of meaninglessness. The third mode he calls moral self-affirmation—the value in a life—and nonbeing threatens moral self-affirmation *relatively* in terms of guilt, and *absolutely* in terms of condemnation. The threat of nonbeing, he says, is constant and gives rise to anxiety related to these six factors of

Existential anxiety results from the threat nonbeing has against self-affirmation.

Existential anxiety is real and has to be experienced.

Modes of self-affirmation	The threat of nonbeing is experienced		Unrealistic demands
	relatively as	absolutely as	
Ontic	*fate*	*death*	Security
Spiritual	*emptiness*	*meaninglessness*	Certitude
Moral	*guilt*	*condemnation*	Perfection

fate and death, emptiness and meaninglessness, guilt and condemnation. Existential anxiety, Tillich states, has an ontological character and cannot be removed. The self has somehow to take this anxiety upon itself, and when it fails to do this, pathological anxiety is the result. Pathological anxiety, in relation to fate and death, produces unrealistic security; in relation to doubt and meaninglessness, produces unrealistic certitude; and in relation to guilt and condemnation, produces unrealistic perfection.

With these three words—security, certitude, and perfection—Tillich has helped us to recognize and understand evil. The truth is that we cannot have absolute security, certainty, or perfection. To want them is understandable, to demand them is diabolical, and to believe that one has already attained them is madness. Evil can readily be found in their pursuit; it is, after all, the pursuit of an illusion nourished by the inability to face reality. Evil can be found not in the ambiguities which pervade human existence, but in people's demand arising from their intolerance of those ambiguities —their demand for security, certitude, and perfection. These demands operate on all the various levels of human experience—global, social, personal.

At the international level the demand for security fosters national self-interest and suspicion of foreigners and reaches its most horrific expression in war. At the social level the demand for security emerges politically in voting for a party on the basis of one's own economic need alone, without regard to other issues of the nation. It is evident in political elitism. Within the church it is expressed in the obstinate refusal to accept change or in simplistic "pie in the sky" religion, which saps one's capacity to question or confront. At the interpersonal level it leads to the debilitating dependency of one person on another or to the seduction or open manipulation of others in order to feel secure. It is illuminating to regard the opposite of love not as hatred but as possessiveness. Hatred at least allows the other his or her separateness and distinctiveness; possessiveness seeks to make the other an extension of oneself. The demand for security is apparent at the psychological level when someone assumes an omnipotent facade, attempts to dominate others, or adopts those superficial world views, whether hedonistic, religious, or pragmatic, which prevent a person from taking risk. At its most horrific it erupts in violence and brutality toward others and in the indifference of those who observe.

At the international level the demand for certitude promotes blatant and narrow nationalism, and even isolation from foreign thought which might be contaminating. At the social level the demand for certitude justifies political cliques, going to the right school, and the criticism of anyone who thinks differently. It lurks in the roots of religious warfare, as well as in the feelings of suspicion or superiority that one religious group, whether Christian or not, has toward another. At the interpersonal level it prevents dialogue and the sharing of ideas and effectively prohibits development of relationships. At the psychological level the demand for certitude sets up barriers to enriching influences from the unconscious mind. Because one cannot be sure where sexual or aggressive drives may lead, they are denied; and when they do emerge, they cannot be integrated into self-awareness. In such circumstances these drives are likely to be unsatisfying to oneself and destructive toward others. The demand for certitude bars surprise from entering and enriching one's life.

At the international level the demand for perfection surfaces in the necessity to be the best— the best oil producer, the best shipbuilder, the best arms manufacturer, the best exporter of natural resources. At the political level those who do not agree are in some way morally degenerate, and this is precisely the thinking that leads to the settling of political disagreements by bloodshed and bullet rather than ballot. At the religious level the demand for perfection leads to spurious experiences of conversion and to the total denial of ambiguity as a reality. At the religious level as well it can be found in the misconception that, by virtue of holding a certain religious office, one is somehow morally elevated above others. At the psychological level the demand for perfection strikes out in the vindictive self-hatred experienced in personal failure, in the single-minded pursuit of success at the expense of family, friends, or anyone who might presume to stand in the way. The demand for perfection is ultimately self-alienating, because we are always faced with the reality of our imperfection.

These are, then, but a few examples of the evil that befalls people in their pathological refusal to accept the reality of their existence—an evil that comes from their demand for security, certitude, and perfection. In this regard, it is of interest to look at the three temptations of Jesus. These temptations could be seen as an attempt to disorient him. In the temptation story the devil appeals to Jesus' desire for security, certitude, and perfection —a desire shared by all humankind. The devil suggested that Jesus use magic to meet his needs. Using magic would give him absolute certainty that he could always have his way, but Jesus did not turn the stones into bread. The devil suggested the way of absolute security, the conquering of nations by force, but Jesus refused to worship the devil. The devil suggested the demonstration of absolute perfection, but Jesus did not cast himself down from the Temple to show that God would save his chosen one. In the temptation story, we see Jesus turn away from the demand for security, certitude, and perfection, and so accept the ambiguity, alienation, and brokenness that life affords.

It was this decision that Dostoevsky's Grand Inquisitor could not accept. The story of the Grand Inquisitor is told by Ivan, one of the Brothers Karamazov, and is the hypothetical account of Jesus' interrogation after he had been imprisoned when he had come again at the time of the Spanish

Inquisition. According to the inquisitor, Jesus could have prevented men and women from having to face the ambiguities of life; he could have taken away their struggles and opted for miracle, mystery, and authority, but he refused to do so. The inquisitor found Jesus guilty of giving people their freedom to struggle and grow, thereby leaving them vulnerable. The challenge of the Grand Inquisitor is echoed by many who proclaim their version of security, certitude, or perfection. One of Tillich's students shows how important this issue was to Tillich and recalls: "The most passionate statement I heard Tillich make in the years I studied with him was that the genuinely prophetic thinkers in the modern age were those who spent a lifetime combating the Grand Inquisitor."[6]

We have argued that the recognition of evil is important in keeping humankind oriented, and we have looked at examples of the greater evil that befalls people when they attempt to deny its presence. In Tillich's terms, it is the threat that nonbeing holds against one's self-affirmation that leads to existential anxiety. It is the attempt to deny and escape this anxiety that leads to the pathological and evil defenses of which we have spoken. Tillich also said that this "existential anxiety . . . cannot be removed but must be taken into the courage to be."[7]

Evil, to be faced, requires courage. The importance of courage in dealing with evil is central to our discussion. It is exciting when theoretical propositions can be demonstrated clinically, and although I cannot present a methodologically sound piece of research on courage, I have been interested in the word for some time, and I often ask the young people I see in my practice what courage is and where it comes from. Often, of course, they give an illustration of courage to clarify their definition. It is interesting how often the illustration they choose shows precisely that quality they need to overcome a major personal difficulty.

A nine-and-a-half-year-old girl was living in considerable stress; she was from a broken home and had twice been in the care of the Children's Aid Society. At the time I saw her, a worker from an agency was coming to the home on a regular basis. This girl was coping with the uncertainty of her life through defiance of authority and constant fighting with her sister. Courage to her was "when you go into the jungle and not be afraid." The jungle of her life, full of shadows and the possibility of sudden and arbitrary attack, was starting to overwhelm her. Courage was required to prevent her from deteriorating into overwhelming anxiety.

A fourteen-and-a-half-year-old girl recounted the most courageous moment of her life. She came from a disturbed family. On Christmas Eve her father, who was an alcoholic, and her brother got into a violent physical fight. The most courageous thing she ever did was "staying there and putting up with it." Courage for this girl enabled her to hold together the fabric of the family for that limited time.

A ten-and-a-half-year-old boy was struggling to deal with the reality of his mother having cancer. He was worried that he too might get sick and die, and he was particularly worried about dying in the night. This, in turn, led to his having trouble sleeping. This boy said that to have courage was to "be brave like you found a lion in the jungle and you don't have a gun and you fought it." He needed courage to fight the lion devouring his mother and, perhaps, him too.

A thirteen-and-a-half-year-old boy, whose parents were divorced and whose mother had just separated from her common-law husband, was in difficulty because he was not working at school, and he was moving with a socially deviant peer group. He seemed to be moving to an increasingly negative opinion of himself. His description of courage was, "You've got to have courage to go on instead of quit." Courage was required for him to continue on the road of his personal growth.

These clinical illustrations show us how courage operates at important points in people's lives—when they can either grow and develop or slip into self-destructive behavior. Courage, whatever else it might be, is the capacity to resist the temptation to demand security, certitude, or perfection—the capacity to face an uncertain and ambiguous reality in which action requires risk. It is apparent that these moments of risk are moments of potential growth and enrichment. This is true no matter at what stage of development a person may be. The application of courage at the point of risk is essential to human growth.

A seven-year-old boy, over several months, was displaying too great a dependence on his mother. He was afraid whenever she went out, although he was left with a capable and familiar sitter. He was becoming increasingly irritable and tantrumous. During this time the child was having a recurrent dream. In the dream, he was near his home when a strange man began to chase him. He would run home, but his legs moved too slowly, and his pursuer gained at each stride. When the child got to the door of his home, he opened it, but his fingers fumbled so that he couldn't shut the door quickly enough to lock it from his pursuer. He would then flee and hide in terror—each time in the same place. The man would hunt for him, opening drawers and cupboards, coming closer and closer to the hiding place, until the boy woke in terror. The dream began to oppress the child so that he thought about it during the day. Finally he resolved to confront this man. The next time he dreamed it, the dream followed the exact pattern to detail, yet even as he ran home and fumbled at the door, he knew what he must do. When the dream had got to the point where he usually awoke in terror, he flung open the door of the cupboard in which he was hiding and thrust out his hand to his pursuer saying, "Hi, how are you?" The pursuer smiled, took his hand, and said, "Fine, how are you?" This dream never recurred, and the child's difficulties soon showed improvement. One can speculate how the child would have developed had he had to flee, hide, and never face his pursuer, but this act of courage moved him forward into a freer life.

A man in his eighties spoke of what he felt had been the most courageous moment in his life. This man had fought in the cavalry during the First World War. He had been wounded. In later years he had faced cancer with its attendant investigations and unpleasant and painful radiation. The most courageous moment for him was when, after completing his professional education and gaining foreign experience, he returned home and, on hearing of a senior position being offered in a company, went directly to the president of the company, to whom he was an absolute unknown, and told him he was the man the president was looking for. At that point this man was risking his self-respect in the profession he loved. Perhaps if he had not risked then, he would have risked later, but one cannot deny the importance of that moment for his life.

We began this discussion by indicating that cooperation between those who sail in the ship of the mind and those who sail in the ship of the soul would lead to a deeper understanding of humankind and to an enrichment of human life. Our dockside conversation has stated that people begin to understand themselves at the point of pain, that much of the pain in their lives is due to the evil that befalls them when they are unable to face the

reality of their lives and, instead, become disoriented through their demands for security, certitude, and perfection, and that a necessary quality
for confronting this evil and, therefore, an essential quality to human growth and enrichment, is
courage.

Courage is, then, a great friend of those who
travel in both ships, and it is a great companion in
the journey of our lives. Our next task will be to
search for the means of attaining it.

2.

Courage Through Covenant

Courage, we have argued, is necessary for dealing with the brokenness, alienation, and ambiguity of human life. Courage operates to move people forward in their own personal growth and development, and is necessary in order for men and women to affirm themselves in spite of the threat of nonbeing. Courage protects people from the growth of illusion; it pushes people into reality. Where courage is lacking, the demand for security, certitude, and perfection grow. Putting this into religious language, we could say that courage gives us the ability to recognize God's creative action in the tension of our lives.

This chapter identifies a major source of courage to be relationship. It will be argued that a central ingredient in the development of courage is the personal experience of relationships based on trust, truth, and clear expectation. Where there are such nourishing relationships, courage will develop, and where there are not, courage will be lacking.

Let us look at how this argument is borne out in a community of people where the matter of relationship was so important that it came to be seen as central to the understanding of reality itself. The ancient Hebrews were a rootless mixture of people. They were people with no memory of land or of ancestral gods; they had no strong blood ties; they were foreigners wherever they went. Some, like Abraham, gained importance and wealth to the point of becoming seminomadic kings, but their influence never endured. In Egypt this collection of people were essentially servants to their Egyptian rulers.

Then something quite remarkable happened. This people gradually began to form together into a community, and they began to confront their oppressors. The courage for this collective self-assertion during this period of confrontation came from their growing sense of unity and self-identity as a people, which in turn was strongly influenced by their growing allegiance to a common God. In the struggles with their oppressors much of their advantage was gained through natural disasters such as infestation and plague. In ancient days such momentous natural occurrences were thought to be weapons of the gods; so their God seemed increasingly powerful to them. When they mustered their courage under the leadership of Moses and overcame their oppressors and escaped, they realized something quite astonishing and impossible had happened. By all that was thought possible, they should never have succeeded, but under the guidance and protection of their God, they did succeed. What a wonder their God has wrought!

It was left to Moses to bring all this experience together into something solid and substantial. It was at Sinai that the profound understanding of covenant occurred. Previously covenants had been set up to form agreements of mutual obligation between individuals or nations. The covenant at Sinai, however, established an agreement between God and his people that was the root of reality itself. To the Hebrew people this radical covenant relationship became the heart of the nation. It was with this vision and understanding that the young nation looked back through its legends and traditions and there identified in retrospect the same quality of covenant. It was after the exodus and Sinai that this covenant relationship was discovered in the stories of Abraham, Isaac, and Jacob. The relationship that gave the people courage to overcome their Egyptian oppressors had earlier given Abraham the courage to "found a nation," and was later to give courage to David as he chose the stones for his sling and went forth to slay the giant enemy warrior.

This quality of covenant relationship was based primarily on trust. Because Abraham trusted in God and agreed to sacrifice his only son, God made his covenant with him. The notion of trust is essential to covenant. A central role of the prophets was to maintain the people's trust in God. They were constantly admonishing their people to hold their faith, faith which was needed to stand in the face of what, at times, appeared to be considerable evidence that God had abandoned his people. The message of the prophets, in this regard, is that people's faith is based on God's trustworthiness— nothing more, nothing less. Faith and duty are closely allied, and for the Hebrew the moral aspect of faith took precedence over the intellectual and emotional aspects. During times when the Lord seemed to be hiding his face (Isa. 8:17) or disregarding people's rights (Isa. 40:27), trust in God gave the Hebrews courage not to fall into resignation and despair. This same trust can be felt in the courageous words that a young Jew wrote on the wall of a Warsaw ghetto, as quoted by Hans Küng: "I believe in the sun, even if it does not shine. I believe in love, even if I do not feel it. I believe in God, even if I do not see him."[8]

At times, however, the people lost trust in their relationship with each other and with their God. It is here that the connecting link between courage and covenant can be demonstrated. When the people lose trust in the covenant or become disoriented from the covenant, they lack the courage to face their existence without demanding security, certitude, and perfection. They seek to satisfy these demands by making their own gods and dominating other lands and people for the sake of their own power. Moreover, when the people are caught in such demands and illusion and are so disoriented, they lack the courage to give up their demands and to put their trust in covenant relationships of trust, truth, and justice. Covenant and courage are mutually supportive and together contribute to sustaining the fabric of community.

The prophet Micah shows how important covenant is for the whole of reality. When the people break covenant, the prophet speaks God's challenge in a court of law. Significantly, the challenge is given before the mountains and hills, and before the enduring foundations of the earth. The whole of reality stands ready to tremble and fall if covenant is broken. The judgment states that because the people have broken the covenant, because they have damaged their relationship with God and each other, they will be faced with social and political upheaval. In religious language this misfortune is interpreted as God's punishment. In sociological and psychological language it can be stated that when relationship is broken, the courage to deal with the ambiguities and uncertainties of life is lost, and the way is then open to all manner of self-interest, social breakdown, and political upheaval.

Let us now speak of covenant more directly from the point of view of psychiatry. Covenant, we have argued, is relationship built on trust, truth, and clear expectation, but as such it is also an important ingredient in mental health. Each of these three elements is essential to healthy relationships. Trust is necessary to hold the relationship together, truth is necessary to maintain productive communication and mutuality of interest, and clear expectation is necessary to keep the relationship on a common course and prevent it from serious disruption and misunderstanding. The three qualities of trust, truth, and clear expectation are necessary to the life of any healthy relationship and are the backbone of any community or society.

Trust could be said to be the primary quality. Abraham's trustworthiness first led God to make covenant with him. It is on the basis of trust that one can then begin to understand the word "truth"—that is to say, without the act of trusting there can be no credence given to truth. Truth becomes rootless or anchorless without trust. The importance of trust is emphasized by Erik Erikson, one of the great psychoanalytic thinkers of the past thirty years. Erikson makes trust a cornerstone in his theory of human development. In his book *Identity and the Life Cycle* he states that the first necessary acquisition on the road to a healthy identification is the establishment of a sense of trust. This is the first step, and according to him the critical period for its acquisition is infancy. This sense of trust, which he refers to as basic trust, must be acquired before children have a sense of autonomous self, and before they have developed the ability to think abstractly. Children's sense of trust is primary even to their idea of self or their capacity to think and understand. One is reminded, from another frame of reference, that faith is primarily a matter of trust rather than intellectual agreement.

Let us look further into Erikson's discussion of

trust. The relationship between mothers and children shows us that infants gain their sense of trust in the relationship not because they move into some power play, but paradoxically because they receive caring and nourishment through their dependency. The infant's weakness and dependency elicit appropriate responses of caring and nourishing from the mother. Trust seems to belong to the natural harmony and resonance of the relationship. Erikson emphasizes the importance of trust growing out of the best possible application of the norms in a particular community. He points out that communities vary; there is no perfect community, but trust will grow when there is an attempt to apply the best direction found in the child's culture. It is in the community struggling to adequately provide for the child that the sense of trust is developed, and not in the appeal to some wondrous and magical new deal.

He writes: "The amount of trust derived from earliest infantile experience does not seem to depend on absolute quantities of food or demonstrations of love but, rather, on the quality of the maternal relationship. Mothers create a sense of trust in their children by that kind of administration which in its quality combines sensitive care of the baby's individual needs and a firm sense of personal trustworthiness within the trusted framework of the community's lifestyle." He goes on to say: "Parents must also be able to represent to a child a deep and almost somatic conviction that there is meaning to what they are doing. In this sense, a traditional system of child care could be said to be a factor making for trust, even when certain items of that tradition, taken singly, may seem irrational or unnecessarily cruel."[9] Trust, in Erikson's terms, grows out of a relationship which has some continuity and endurance to it.

This sense of trust continues through life, it is informed and not contradicted by intellect and understanding, and it is integral to relationships of intimacy. Trust works to preserve relationships through those periods of conflict which will always occur if a relationship is to move forward into greater depths. Trust, then, is not some empty-headed, ephemeral, or blind affiliation to something but a basic quality necessary to personal growth. Trust, in a sense, is the crystal around which the rest of the personality solidifies.

We live in a world where even the most intimate relationships are still incomplete, and there is nothing more destructive of a relationship than a pervading sense of mistrust. Mistrust leads us to approach others with suspicion and hide our real intentions, paving the way to confusing and bewildering transactions. Mistrust prompts us to pull rank on another lest he or she unseat us with a clever remark or shatter the illusion of our power by pointing out that we, like the emperor, have no clothes. Mistrust moves us to employ seduction to gain our ends, because we fear a straightforward request will mean our rejection. Mistrust of others leads to our personal isolation in which we are unwilling to say where our hurts really are, for fear that they will become a target for further attack. Most tragic of all, mistrust of ourselves leaves us uncertain and bewildered, caught between moving forward into the reality of life or fleeing headlong into resignation and despair. It is here that our understanding of covenant reaches our daily lives. God reaches out in his love to his people; a mother reaches out in love to her child. In these covenants we find trust, and in this trust we find courage to face our lives. In the experience of God's covenant we glimpse the eternal quality of a mother's act of love, and in our experience of a mother's love we glimpse the depth of the love of God.

Truth is a second element of covenant which can help us in our quest for courage. For our purposes, telling the truth means being as honest as possible within the context of a given situation. Speaking the truth can really not be separated from the context of the telling. Communications theory talks of a meta-communication, which is a communication about the communication. There is no such thing as telling the truth in the abstract; it always happens in the context of a relationship. If a child is told by a child-welfare worker that his or her mother has been put in jail, the child is not only getting information at a verbal level about the mother, but is also being told at the nonverbal level that this world is full of sudden, seemingly arbitrary events that one learns about from strangers. We cannot tell one truth without behaving another truth. Here again the primacy of trust is demonstrated. In a sense it could be said that the truth can never be heard from an untrusted person.

The healing power of truth and the importance of trust is illustrated in the following example of a child-welfare worker who was worried about a child of six living in a lie. This child was staying with two older brothers in a foster home. Her father, who was in a mental hospital, had, when in a disturbed state, murdered the children's mother. The older two children had witnessed this, but the child, who was just a toddler at the time, had been asleep and had no memory of the event and had been kept from the truth. This sensitive worker realized the growing isolation of the child and the danger implicit in her hearing the facts suddenly or brutally later in life, when she would be alone and unsupported. The worker, after painstakingly planning how the event of telling the truth could be structured, approached the foster parents for their help, because she knew that she must have the parents present to support the child. It was arranged with the foster parents, and on the day of the telling the worker spoke to the older brothers, explained what she was going to do, and asked whether they would come in while the event took place. They at first refused but then agreed. The worker began by telling the child the dreadful truth in as simple and honest a way as she possibly could, and before she was through she was interrupted by the older brothers, who through their tears, completed the story. The child asked why her brothers were crying, and in that question began to accept the truth of what had been a hidden part of her life. This is a beautiful illustration of truth told in the context of trust. The worker had labored long and hard in structuring the event of the telling, but what she could never have programmed was the spontaneous and healing behavior of the older brothers, who spoke and behaved the truth so beautifully and, in so doing, set their sister free from the prison of silence in which she had lived. The courage of this worker enabled the child to learn the truth in a relationship of trust and so gain the courage to take a step forward into the reality of her own life.

This example of truth-telling can be contrasted to Ibsen's play *The Wild Duck,* in which truth was told insensitively and out of context. The play shows how when truth is told from a presumptuous position of power, it becomes destructive. In the play the hasty declaration of a family secret leads to the tragic death of the only child in the family. Truth brandished insensitively and hastily becomes in effect a lie, because it distorts the truth. The evil in such a situation is the teller's illusion of power and certitude in the telling. The teller must acknowledge the relativity, uncertainty, and incompleteness of the context in which he speaks, and he must see the person to whom he is talking, not as an object to suit his ends, but as a fellow traveler and a brother or sister who has to be taken seriously.

There continues to exist a simplistic notion that

as long as we tell the truth everything is all right. To have an affair with another man will not matter if I tell my husband. To think another woman more attractive than my wife is fine as long as I let her know. The telling may be factual, but the real message is one of hostile manipulation. The factual truth will likely be destructive when there is no trust in the relationship. Perhaps the line that best sums up the emptiness of a relationship of truth without trust is the caption of a cartoon which reads, "Let's face it, Sarah, our analyzing the basis of our relationship is the foundation of our relationship."

When there is both trust and truth, we are able to set realistic expectations for ourselves and for our relationships. Whether we are aware of it or not, we always expect something from a relationship. Accurate and realistic expectations build relationships, while presumptuous and unrealistic expectations destroy relationships. Great friendships and intimate relationships are built on clear understanding of what each expects of the other. The better one knows the other, the more one knows what to expect. The same is true in therapeutic relationships—the more the expectation for therapist and client is clear and mutually agreed on, the more the relationship is likely to be functional and healing. This, of course, acknowledges that relationships are always undergoing some change, and that new expectations may emerge as the relationship develops.

In contrast, when expectations are unclear or

unilateral they are likely to be destructive of the relationship. If we alter Charles Dickens' title from *Great Expectations* to *Unrealistic Expectations,* we can add the subtitle *The Destroyer of Community.* We may, for example, set unrealistic expectations for what a government will be able to achieve. We do not accurately assess the facts of the situation, and we hide from the problems of the nation. But in our demand for security we are unrealistic. In holding false expectations, we at the same time abdicate our own responsibility in working toward change. When the government fails, and fail it must in a climate of unreal expectation, we respond in anger and criticism. Our passions may lead some of us into simplistic solutions of anarchy and revolution or, conversely, into apathy and withdrawal. The healthy response is to examine our initial expectation and then to bring it as close to the facts as we possibly can.

Unrealistic expectations often flourish in the life of the church. As the Grand Inquisitor points out, people want to be taken care of and be free of their burdens. Because these people profess to be believers, they also expect, in some marvelous way, that God will end their struggle. When life continues to be problematic and burdensome, those who hold this unrealistic expectation are cast into doubt and despair. In the same vein, people often expect the clergy to be special Christians and consequently may hold them responsible for any faults in a parish. The clergy, on their part, can be caught up in the flattery of exaggerated expectation and take on more than they can effectively perform. In the absence of clear expectations, responsibilities can accumulate and the relationship collapse into mutual hostility or resignation.

Similar problems exist for mental health professionals. People who come for help often expect to be given freedom from pain and struggle. Help in this sense would mean the remaking of reality itself. If this unrealistic expectation is allowed to persist, then the assessment and advice of the mental health professional will never be adequate, and the patient will go away more alienated and embittered with life than before.

Another word for forming clear expectations has been "contracting." This is especially important when we are involved in a helping relationship. Contracting involves a clear working out of what each person expects from the relationship and agrees to do within the relationship. Contracting ensures an active listening to the other's expectation, as well as a clear statement of one's own expectation, until a mutual agreement is found.

To neglect such social contracting is to open the door to manipulation, however unconscious such manipulation might be. One kind and well-meaning clergyman, who had good reason to expect to become wealthy, decided he would give his services free to a poor and needy parish. On the surface this might appear to be a creative and useful endeavor. What he overlooked in this proposal was that he was assuming a position of power in the parish, because those who were not paying him would have little stomach to challenge him at any point. By not attempting to consult the people about the nature of their future relationship, he was really saying that in his ministry arbitrary power plays would be a strong possibility. It appeared that in his ministry he would be a giver and they would be receivers, and there would be no mutual endeavors.

Unrealistic expectations are particularly destructive in marriage. Marriage continues to be romanticized in our culture to the extent that there is a spurious, mythical, "happy ever afterward" aura about it. Marriage does not insulate people from the brokenness of the world. Marriage cannot protect a person from the attack of an employer, ineffective office interaction, or a drop in the economy. Yet often there is an implicit message to the spouse to make it better. The exaggerated demands on the marriage only lead to its destruction. A common mistake of would-be helpers is to make assumptions about what is wrong with a marriage without really mustering the facts and without searching out the expectations of each for the other. This is a common flaw in many of the so-called "sex therapies." The assumption is made that if the couple's sex life improves, their marriage will improve. This is at best a short-term solution. It may distract the couple from their alienation, but unless they are able actually to face their unrealistic expectations for each other, they will continue to erode and destroy the relationship.

Unrealistic expectations are also destructive in parenting. All parents have to struggle to know and love their child as he or she really is. The unrealistic expectations usually take root in some personal need of the parent. Worldly success and achievement, both of which are so highly rated in our culture, implicitly require that the successful parent have a successful child. If the parents are to live with their real child, they must put to death and mourn the false image they have created. When they give up the demand that their child be secure and perfect, they turn to meet the real person that is their child. Parents of children who are physically handicapped or mentally impaired have the task of mourning and burying their ideal child each time they become aware of the contrast between their child and what he or she might have been. It is in this simple acceptance of reality that they find intimacy with their child.

An example of how unrealistic expectations are destructive in a parent-child relationship can be shown in the demand that the child always tell the truth. What is overlooked is that there is a deeper aspect to the relationship, and this is trust. Children do not tell the truth when, for some reason, they cannot trust the relationship. Lack of trust may stem from fear of the parents, from a low opinion of themselves, or from some kind of external stress in the relationship. Whatever the cause, wise parents recognize that when their children lie, they are also saying that they are unable to trust the present situation with the truth. If the parents move in a hostile and heavy fashion to attack the lie, they at the same time increase the children's mistrust. In this way the parents not only weaken their relationship with the children but they also make it more likely that the children will lie again.

I would like to stretch the analogy of covenant from the example of politics, religion, and the interpersonal relationships of marriage and parenting, to include the intrapsychic relationship between the unconscious and the conscious mind. (I realize there is still a necessity in some circles to defend the existence of the unconscious mind, but we have not the time to reopen that particular debate.) To paraphrase Carl Jung, writing in his last book, *Man and His Symbols,* humankind is doomed unless people can open themselves to their unconscious mind.[10] A particularly powerful aspect of Jung's understanding of the unconscious is that, like the biblical idea of covenant, the unconscious links people with the whole of their history and tradition. Yet from the unconscious, with its anchors in the past, fresh insights come, new life springs, and creativity erupts. When we learn to trust our unconscious, we can be surprised by life, we can be shaken to our foundations, and we can be made new again.

Material in the unconscious is beyond conscious control and so can be threatening to those who demand security, certitude, and perfection, who then do their best to fight it and ignore it. They may imprison themselves in compulsive behavior or adopt an authoritarian and regimented lifestyle. They discredit the everyday expressions of unconscious activity—daydreams, hunches, slips of the tongue—and avoid reflection or meditation. If they do happen to remember a dream, they are embarrassed by its sexual content, afraid of its aggressive content, and disgusted by its morbid content, and they try to forget it or shrug it off. Above all, they refuse to see that somehow the dream holds a truth of their life, a truth that might refresh them or help them in an important decision.

We might do well to make a covenant with our unconscious minds. This could be a covenant of peace and respect in which we agree to love and cherish the unconscious, to listen to it and attempt to move as it directs, to the extent that our reason, intellect, and compassion allow. In response our unconscious might well continue to nourish us, surprise us, enrich us, and put breath into our otherwise lifeless bodies.

We have sought courage, the courage to face reality and to give up the demand for security, certitude, and perfection, and we have found it living in covenant. It is not surprising that the church can refer to the wine at the Eucharist as the blood of the new covenant, for that person whose blood was shed for us lived courageously with complete trust and in total truth, and his relationships with his fellow men and women were all clear, straightforward, and without deception.

Courage continues to live in the covenant that gives us trust in life, allows us to speak the truth, and binds us into relationships of clear and mutual expectation.

3.
Meaning Through Symbol

We have stated that if we are to live in freedom we must acknowledge the reality of evil and in our own lives perceive and confront the evil that is before us and within us. We have further argued that courage is necessary for both this perception and confrontation. Our argument until now has been based on elements from human experience and relationship. Evil is found in the experience of human life, and courage grows out of the covenant relationships in that experience. Experience and relationship are, however, not sufficient in themselves for a lifetime of combat with the Grand Inquisitor, for he cannot be overcome by dint of sheer courage and defiance, as important as these are. He must also be met with words—words that are the substance and distillation of human reason, intellect, and understanding.

The Judeo-Christian tradition has always held reason to be essential to faith, in the sense that valid belief is not held by suspending reason or in contradiction to reason but in maintaining harmony with reason. We have already stated that trust in the basic relationships of life and the capacity for self-affirmation are formed in the child before the development of reason. However, when reason does develop, it tends to inform this trust rather than contradict it.

For us to have peace of mind, life has to make sense to us. At times, it is a very great struggle for us to make sense of things, and all too often we are in the darkness of confusion. There is, however, no place for the abandonment of reason. In fact, it is in circumstances which seem inaccessible to our understanding that we are profoundly alienated from self and from others. While courage is necessary to confront the reality of our lives, reason and understanding are necessary to illuminate this reality.

Those who practice psychotherapy, or who are active in helping people in difficulty or trouble, will be familiar with the very powerful effect that moments of such illumination can have. Into the chaos and confusion of broken lives and troubled relationship comes a glimmer of understanding, and something at last makes sense. Such illumination may not alter the actual antagonism or alienation, but into the despair of what seems to be puzzling, brutal, and incomprehensible has come the possibility of meaning. Such illumination may take place within the relationships of marriage or family, or within the people themselves. It is when we are caught in confusion and meaninglessness that we tend to feel most alone and vulnerable. The

Judeo-Christian position asserts that we are never alone in that God is present with us. We must somehow come to grips with this fact and incorporate it into our identity. The relationship with God must be seen to touch all levels of our existence— our nation, our community, our families, and ourselves. It is the task of each new generation of theologians to search for appropriate language to demonstrate this relationship between God and humanity and so to illuminate the lives of people in every age.

Our attempt to understand ourselves and our world has always led us to discover symbols that help capture the truth and spirit of the time. A symbol, however, must do more than capture the present truth; it must somehow look beyond itself and, therefore, act as a guide as well as a source of nourishment. A symbol, if it is to grasp the hearts and spirits of men and women, must reach through the norms, constraints, and legalities of their culture. In so doing, it must compete with the cultural forces that are self-serving and demanding of security, certitude, and perfection. A symbol, if it is to grasp the heart and spirit, must be nourished by that which expresses the depth of the human condition at each time in history. A symbol is not a static, lifeless entity but a dynamic force that emerges from and blends with the life, understanding, and history of a people. This is true for a particular symbol that may be useful to an individual as well as for a collective symbol that may influence the community or nation. Symbols can either inspire people or imprison them; they can open people into life or can shut them into pursuits of power or self-aggrandizement.

Rollo May points to the importance of symbol by noting that cultures collapse when their symbols are no longer useful (can no longer be integrated into the peoples' lives), and people cannot find other symbols to replace them.[11] He also states that we live in an age in need of new symbols. Certainly a quick look at our North American culture does not give us any cause to disagree with him. In a search for present-day symbols, we all might come up with different suggestions, but an event that would seem to model much of what passes for symbol in current North American culture is the Superbowl. The Superbowl pulls together the culturally heralded qualities of combat, strength, and technique, and points toward some sense of future victory and accomplishment. But it is an empty and debilitating symbol, for the victory is ephemeral and vicarious and of no enduring benefit.

Rollo May would seem to be right; we are in need of new symbols. The central point of this chapter is that within our Judeo-Christian heritage there lies a wealth of history and tradition, and that from this rich source events can be brought forward into the present, to become symbols that can give meaning to our lives. Before carrying the discussion further and choosing certain events, we need to make three statements by way of background.

The first background observation reminds us that change is an essential part of reality. Change permeates all the natural order and is, of course, a fundamental factor in human life. The show advertisement that proclaims, "You will never be the same after seeing this thrilling performance," is true as far as it goes, but what it leaves out is, "You will never be the same if you don't see this thrilling performance." We are never the same; we are always changing. The realization of the essential nature of change often causes emotional discomfort that, at certain times of crisis and most obviously in situations of death and dying, may be temporarily debilitating. The relentless march of years can be seen in our faces and felt in our joints. Astronomers tell us that nothing remains the same; even old faithful Polaris, the North Star, is moving. Our own galaxy is itself revolving and makes one revolution in about two hundred million years, which means that since the exodus, by rough calculation, our galaxy has traveled 1/58,000 of a revolution. Our own planet makes its annual rotation around the sun in one brief year. On our planet the monarch butterfly goes through seven generations in its travel from southern to northern habitat. Change and time have always fascinated human beings, but where we can go wrong is in pretending that we can somehow prevent change. Grasping power in the attempt to make something permanent, or to make some indelible mark on history, is folly. Those who avoid the reality of change, by thinking that they "have it made," are misled and are opting out of reality into the illusion of permanence or power.

The desire for permanence is perhaps most poignant in the matter of relationship. Yet all our relationships undergo change. We can never capture a relationship and hold on to it or freeze it; it is always moving. The loving couple who one day think they have reached the point of final understanding together are bewildered, or perhaps shaken, to find themselves struggling in misunderstanding a week or two later, or perhaps even the same evening. We cannot stop change by cants or by cosmetics; it is part of our reality. If we are to live richly, we must face change and integrate it into our lives.

The second background observation is that characteristically human beings look for meaning in the events and circumstances of their lives. When misfortune befalls, people commonly ask, Why did it have to happen? or Why me? Part of the reason people review and re-review tragic events is to uncover some clue, some key, or some theme that will help them make sense out of the bewilderment they find themselves in. The fatalist might be critical of such struggles for understanding, but, after all, a fatalistic outlook is the simplistic avoidance of reality. It is an attempt to accept life through nonengagement. This avoidance of reality may be contrasted with Viktor Frankl's observations about his life in a Nazi concentration camp. He wrote of the horror of these camps, the brutality and the death. Out of this experience he chose the title *A Man's Search for Meaning.* Among many of the moving passages in the book is a brief section in which he talks to his fellow inmates about the meaning of their existence. There, in the cramped and smelly hut, these men were separated from their loved ones and their futures and were aware that they would likely soon be dead.

He writes of how he tried to help them gain perspective by showing how, even then, their situation was not the most terrible they could think of. He spoke of the future and their awareness of the small chance for survival. He spoke also of the past and its joys. He continues: "Then I spoke of the many opportunities of giving life a meaning. I told my comrades (who lay motionless although occasionally a sigh could be heard) that human life, under any circumstances, never ceases to have a meaning, and that this infinite meaning of life includes suffering and dying, privation and death. I asked the poor creatures who listened to me attentively in the darkness of the hut to face up to the seriousness of our position. They must not lose hope but should keep their courage in the certainty that the hopelessness of our struggle did not detract from its dignity and its meaning."[12] His efforts were rewarded by the tears of gratitude in the eyes of those who came to offer him thanks. In this book, Frankl makes the point that the prisoners who had the capacity to go on and not be overwhelmed by apathy and despair were those who had a sense of purpose in their lives. The search for meaning is not, however, the task of the incarcerated and victimized only; it is also the task of the free and productive—the task of every person. It is as important for those who feel they live ordinary and unspectacular lives to come to some sense of the meaning of their lives as it is for those who have achieved some apparent fame and notoriety or find themselves in the center of important world events or catastrophes.

One of the great tasks of the poet, playwright, novelist, and artist is to look at life and give it meaning. Imparting meaning to a human life does not provide any immediate practical benefit, it does not add a cubit to a person's stature, but it does provide a perspective for one's vision, a context for one's self-understanding, and a purpose for one's self-affirmation.

The third background observation is that biography can be theology. McClendon's book *Biography as Theology* presents the thesis that individual human lives can be the expression of theological themes and principles.[13] He writes that people with some degree of consciousness may live out theological themes in their lives. Dag Hammarskjöld understood himself as Christ's brother, and as brother to brother he saw the significance of his life as a sacrifice to be offered. Martin Luther King understood his work under the image of the exodus; he was leading his people on a new crossing of the Red Sea; he was a Moses who went to the mountaintop but was not privileged to enter with his people into the Promised Land.

It is, however, not only the biographies of the

famous, but also the biography of every man and woman, that can become theology. One way of talking about this is to use the notion of journey— a poetic reference to biography. Herbert O'Driscoll describes four journeys in human life.[14] The *first* journey is the outward journey that may be seen by an observer—including work, the social role, possessions, and so on. The *second* journey is the inward journey into the mind, the emotions, and thought. The *third* journey, which, he says, is perhaps the most troublesome but rewarding, is the journey into human relationships. The *fourth* journey begins when we ask the meaning of the other three journeys, and this is the religious journey. He makes the point that storytelling has always been a vehicle for the proclamation of great truths about humankind. The great stories from our Judeo-Christian heritage, he argues, are not simply to be read as ancient history, but are to be used as refreshing insights into our present circumstance. He quite simply states, "We must make the story our story." The religious quest begins at the point of meaning; religion serves mental health when it can help people find meaning. Religion is abused, as are the people it affects, when it is used to turn people away from themselves into magic and pretense.

At this point we are ready to return to the focus of our present discussion, which is to look at the possibility of finding meaning in life through the use of symbol. Four realities are chosen as symbols for that purpose. These fourfold realities come from the heart of our tradition—Bethlehem, Gethsemane, Calvary, and the open tomb. They are the events of the incarnation, the struggle in the Garden, the death on the cross, and the resurrection. These four keystone events can function as symbols and can help people to see the events of their lives in the context of a larger, deeper, and more meaningful reality. Symbols can be reflected upon and thought about in a seemingly infinite number of ways.

Incarnation holds many truths for humankind, and among these the incarnation speaks of the importance of human life. In religious terms, God indicates through the incarnation the value that he puts on human nature. Although God is incarnate in all of his creation, at the nativity of Jesus he became incarnate in a particular way—God himself became a human being in all ways like ourselves.

In discussing the prologue to John, Rudolf Bultmann explains that in our longing we erect an illusion of God. We expect the Revealer "as a shining, mysterious, fascinating figure, as a hero or as a miracle worker or mystagogue. His humanity is to be no more than a disguise; it must be transparent. Men want to look away from the humanity and see and sense the divinity, they want to penetrate the disguise—or they will expect the humanity to be no more than the visualization or the form of the divine." This, in Bultmann's words, is the stuff of illusion. He goes on: "All such desires are cut short by the statement: The Word became flesh. It is in his sheer humanity that he is the revealer." He goes on: "Doxa [glory] is not to be seen *alongside* the sarx [flesh], nor *through* the sarx as through a window; it is to be seen in the sarx and nowhere else. If man wants to see the doxa, then it is upon the sarx he must concentrate his attention."[15] The sarx, the flesh, is not mere trapping, but is essential to the human understanding of God. Incarnation, then, affirms human nature and leads each person to recognize that he or she is significant simply by being alive and human.

Gethsemane speaks of the reality of ambiguity and uncertainty in life. Here Jesus struggled with thoughts of personal freedom and safety, and the principles of love, truth, and justice that he espoused. Every human being will face confusion, bewilderment, and fear, and Gethsemane says that in such circumstances one need not feel guilty, impotent, or stupid. Growth and completeness depend on our confronting the void and not on our pretending that it will disappear. Gethsemane reminds us that if we are to have freedom, we must also face ambiguity and uncertainty; where there is no choice, there is no freedom.

Calvary speaks the truth that if people live honestly and in love, they are bound to suffer and experience death. Jesus remained true to himself and his principles, and at Calvary he was crucified as a traitor. Dying is experienced not only in corporal death but also in the death of relationships, and in the death of visions in the face of harsh realities. Calvary says that death is not shameful or ignoble. Worldly power and success are not essential to what is whole and complete, because there on the cross, in total impotence, was fulfilled the most perfect and complete expression of human life ever lived.

Resurrection speaks of new life arising from death. On the first Easter the friends and followers of Jesus came to the surprising realization that all of what he represented was not dead but alive. Gethsemane informs us that if we live completely, struggle is inevitable; Calvary tells us that death is inevitable; resurrection tells us, when the struggle is begun and death is faced, that the emergence of something new and creative is inevitable. It is in this covenant of resurrection that we find hope and courage to face all our Gethsemanes and Calvaries.

These symbols emerge in all aspects of life—incarnation in creating new and renewed friendship or new vocational possibilities; Gethsemane in struggling to make decisions in contradictory and ambiguous situations; crucifixion in facing the impact of painful events or dreadful realities; and resurrection in opening to new richness of love and friendship, and new depths of perspective and understanding. There is nothing presumptuous in matching these symbols with events in our own lives; there is no confusing of ourselves with Jesus. Instead, we are affirming our belief in the significance and healing power of these great symbolic events.

These symbols may be seen in many dimensions

of human life. In the process of thought one speaks of the idea incarnate, the ideal assailed by criticism and doubt, the pain of recognizing error and fault, and finally the resurrection of a new and more encompassing truth. In the growth of relationship, one speaks of the birth or meeting with all its attendant excitement and possibility; the tumult of the forces of indifference and uncertainty, the pain of the death of an imagined, ideal friendship, and the emergence of a truer and more intimate relationship. Human life itself encompasses birth, the struggling for identity and integrity, the pain of recognizing and facing death, and the feeling of having lived with meaning and purpose.

Everyone at times arrives in Gethsemane. The business executive at a meeting torn with indecision; the youth trying to decide what to do with his or her life, realizing one choice precludes another; the lover, unable to make a commitment because of uncertainty or the fear of being limited; the person poised yet frozen at the point of decision, aware of innumerable pros and cons and feeling crushed between the demand for action and the lack of certainty—all these are in Gethsemane. The recognition of this symbol might help free them from the profound sense of despair and alienation that is often part of such moments.

The resolution of Gethsemane is found at Calvary. The confusion of depression gains clarification in the painful awareness of what is really wrong with one's life, and this awareness is the beginning of possible change. An illustration of this point is provided by the experience of one partner in a marriage. He had been complaining that something was wrong, that his marriage wasn't as it should be, and that he was honestly struggling to improve it. In a particularly painful argument, his wife was finally able to show him how he had kept her boxed into a certain category, and because of this she couldn't be what he wanted. This realization brought enormous pain and sadness to him, over what he had done and what had been missed, but at this moment the relationship became stronger and more loving than it had ever been. His confusion was lifted, but it had taken its toll; nevertheless, he had grown into a relationship he hadn't thought possible.

It will be apparent that each resurrection is in another sense a new incarnation. The idea that emerges as a new and more encompassing truth will once again be subjected to criticism. The relationship that emerges from conflict into greater love and intimacy will once again enter conflict. A person who has gained a sense of meaning and purpose in life will continue to search through confusion and apparent absurdity. These symbols, far from being a stagnating influence, help people to accept and move with change.

These symbols relate to the ongoing events of life in a continuous, cyclical pattern. If this pattern is interrupted, difficulties emerge. The progression can stop at any of the four stages. Incarnation may fail to move forward into Gethsemane. This happens, for example, when people succumb to the narcissism of indulging their own perceptions or sensations, or spend excessive energy in imagining future glories and success, or adopt a world view that holds difficulty and suffering to be alien to proper living and to be avoided at all cost, or allow the wonder and excitement of sexual experience to become an end in itself without care for others involved.

The progression may also stop at Gethsemane and not move forward to Calvary. Such is the case when people, with reduced tolerance to ambiguity, become caught in depression and confusion. They long for security, perfection, and certainty, the longing tends to become a demand, and the situation deteriorates with the growing frustration of not having these demands met. Psychological relief in such situations may be obtained by certain mental maneuvers, many of which occur outside awareness. These involve projecting the cause of one's difficulties on to others so that the blame falls elsewhere, turning away one's emotional involvement so that things don't really matter, or distorting the events so that the situation becomes more palatable at the price of breaking with reality. The mental health professional could use the words "paranoia," "neurosis," and "psychosis" in reference to these phenomena, but whatever the language, their crippling effect is the same.

Another more conscious maneuver is to grasp at straws thrown by some expert who presumes to have the solution and the special way around Calvary. Religion is, at times, responsible for seducing people to avoid Calvary. This is the more reprehensible when the initial contact is made with the people in their Gethsemanes. The preacher is aware of people's loneliness, confusion, and despair, and his or her voice flows through the radio or television: "There may be some of you out there hearing my voice this very moment who feel this hurt or that kind of bewilderment." Then, however, the preacher does not endorse these feelings as proper to human experience, but just the opposite. The next step suggests that Jesus can take them all away. Converts meet the Savior in Gethsemane and magically escape Calvary. The solution appeals to their dependency and longing for significance. They are introduced into an antiseptic world that, as this word implies, is lifeless. While they may feel some sense of relief, they have stopped encountering reality. They are now somehow insulated from evil and free from the dilemma of ambiguity. Cares and worries become sinful and reflect moral weakness. Instead of being faced, they are wondrously laid aside. Calvary has been avoided. Any psychological energy that might serve to criticize what is happening to them is channeled into arguing with opponents or gaining new converts—practices that serve to reassure them that they are on track. (One cannot help wondering what would happen to this energy if there were no unbelievers left to convert.)

It is not, however, only this particular brand of Christianity that offers a way around Calvary. Experts are always available to direct people to a pain- and tension-free existence. They often assume a traditional healing or religious role, or ride the crest of some new fad. Whatever the guise of the helpers, it is unlikely that they will be of any real help unless they are able to point the person out of Gethsemane toward Calvary. There is no avoiding the reality that if we choose to do one thing, we cannot do another. When a girl chooses between two men, she hurts one. There is no escaping the fact that in this broken world every act has a destructive as well as constructive edge. Human action is imperfect and incomplete and necessarily carries with it an element of destructiveness. It is when destructiveness is faced, rather than denied, that there can be some reparation. But there is no chance for healing when behavior that has been hurtful or confusing to others is rationalized away as being "unimportant," "unavoidable," or "the way it goes." Helping a person move forward from Gethsemane is likely to mean helping the person face, and then reject, illusions of insulation and protection from reality, as well as helping the person nourish a capacity for relationship with friends, family, and community which will in turn give the courage necessary to move forward.

The progression may also stop at Calvary, where in the pain of real or apparent failure, there is no comprehension of the opportunities made available through the action taken. Sorrow can be unduly prolonged and can become the source of petulance and meanness. The person, in an inability to see any accomplishment in what he or she has done, becomes increasingly self-critical or vindictive toward others.

Resurrection, instead of becoming the springboard to newness, may stop in prolonged self-congratulation or in the illusion that all has now been accomplished. If excessive self-indulgence develops, there will be no room left for openness to further criticism and refinement. Movement is required if one is to live in reality. There is, in fact, no rest from the cycle of these four themes through our lives. This was well expressed in these words taken from a sermon preached about the office for the burial of the dead: "Jesus saw life as haunted by an extraordinary urgency as though the Kingdom of God is always to be found around the next bend in the road . . . just a few more steps and you will be there, sobbing with relief, joy, and the consciousness of being forgiven. Yet he also sees the mistaken choices and destructive decisions we make in our longing for that joy. He tries to persuade us to relax the tension of that search and to have one care only . . . the longing for God."[16] Life, to be lived in health, must be lived in urgency.

We have talked of finding meaning through symbol. An important work of the biographer is to take a person's life and give it meaning by setting it into a context or background that makes it informative and interesting. The fourfold symbols of incarnation, Gethsemane, crucifixion, and resurrection could be looked on as a context and background for each and every human life—a larger context and background into which the biographer could set the more personal biographical facts. The richness of life, in whatever circumstance of obscurity or notoriety, might well be measured not by worldly success, prestige, or power but by the degree to which this life was alive with the constant movement of these four eternal, symbolic themes.

4.
Salvation Through Suffering

We have recognized that evil is a reality of our existence and have found the courage to face evil through relationships of truth, trust, and justice. We have sought meaning for our lives through the fourfold symbols of incarnation, Gethsemane, crucifixion, and resurrection. We have discovered these truths, and with them all we remain at the threshold of our new history. At each moment we must step forward, making the history that is our lives, and it is in the making of this history that we find our salvation. But this history belongs to an imperfect and limited creature—a creature who must step forward knowing that while evil is recognized, it continues present and powerful; while courage is available, it emerges through relationships that are uncertain and incomplete; and while meaning is clarifying and energizing, it remains threaded with ambiguity. If it is by stepping forward into life that we walk toward salvation, then an essential companion on our journey will be suffering.

The central argument of this chapter is that suffering is an essential component in human salvation. Suffering and salvation are both emotionally charged words and so have the capacity to bring into our minds a host of images. Suffering, in the sense it is used here, is the experience and appreciation of the alienation and incompleteness of the human condition. Suffering is found in our finiteness, our imperfection, and our incompleteness. Suffering, in this sense, is both a cognitive and an emotional experience: it involves both thought and feeling and is also related to, but distinct from, frustration and pain. Suffering, then, is not being seen as a gradient of pain (in the way that severe pain is called suffering and can be contrasted to mild pain or discomfort). Nor should suffering ever be understood, through a perverted sense of virtue, as something pleasurable or something to be sought. People can never like to suffer. Suffering is an experience essential to human salvation because it is a natural component of the confrontation with reality. It is in meeting reality, and not turning away from it, that people find both their suffering and their salvation.

The vision of what life may be leads us to suffer when we look at our present situation. The vision of what life might have been leads us to suffer when we see orphaned children, no matter how successful, content, or happy they might appear to be; when we see a marriage end in divorce, no matter how constructive and needed the divorce might be; when we see the poor in their confusion, impotence, and apathy. Such is the stuff of human suffering. When we are unable to acknowledge suffering, we do not show our insensitivity to the pain and tragedy of human life as much as we show our lack of vision of what human life ought to be or might become.

It is proper for the historian to catalog and understand the tumultuous events in the life of nations; it is helpful for the psychoanalyst to sort out how events and dynamics in lives contribute to the present emotion and behavior of those in his or her care; it is constructive for the politician to perceive human need and to act to meet it. Historians, analysts, politicians, and men and women of learning from many other pursuits catalog, comment on, and help to remedy the problems and inadequacies of the human condition, but the insight and eloquence of such experts, however helpful they might be, should never insulate us against the suffering that permeates the stuff of their work.

Suffering functions much like a homing device that keeps us heading into the reality of our existence and prevents us from spinning off track into some diversion, whether it be hedonistic, rationalistic, or spiritualistic. The point that suffering can be likened to a homing device is illustrated by the experience of one twelve-year-old girl. This girl had been through difficult times at home. Her father was ill, and her mother's energies were given to her husband and to her son, who was a great problem for the family. The girl matured early sexually and was teased unmercifully at school.

She was a lonely and isolated child. Her great comfort and gift was her own brilliant and imaginative mind; she enjoyed literature, music, and the arts. In her loneliness she would often long just to disappear into her daydreams. She had a favorite daydream in which she would be in a beautiful meadow lying on the grass and gazing into the beautiful blue sky. While lying there she felt utterly content and free, and she would want to stay there forever. Always, however, some dreadful wild animal would come into the dream and scare her back into the reality of her waking life. This story reminds us that what at first appears pleasant may be drawing us into illusion, and that what startles us back to reality may later serve to promote growth and healing. This young girl's experience reminds us that peacefulness and escape cannot be permanent.

Turning this point slightly, we could liken suffering to the quality of restlessness that Augustine speaks of in the powerful statement, "You made us for yourself and our hearts find no peace until they rest in you."[17] It seems that, although we may find moments of joy, recreation, refreshment, and even repose, our hearts still remain restless in our onward-moving historical struggle—of such is suffering and in such is salvation.

Salvation is a central theme in any theology. It could even be argued that the underlying motivation for people to think theologically is their realization that they need to be saved from sin or, using other language, to be set free from that within them which demands unreality and so leads to disorientation and isolation. In people's need to be saved, they are moved to wonder about God and his action. When the sense of sin eventually emerges through all the defenses that people build up against it, they see their brokenness and alienation and look for salvation. Salvation, however, is found not by moving out of their worldly circumstance but by moving more thoroughly and deeply in to it.

Salvation in Western tradition has always been linked to history. We may remind ourselves that it was the mighty acts of God in the history of his people that were finally recognized in the covenant at Sinai. This rooting of salvation in actual events is what so sharply distinguishes the biblical doctrine of salvation from other theologies. The Jewish people are reminded of the reality and power of God not through any theory or set of ideas, not through a logical deduction from a theistic philosophy, nor yet through any technique of mystical absorption with the divine, but by remembrance and recognition of his acts in history.[18] The prophets constantly draw the people back to the reality of God's action in their history. The biblical doctrine of salvation is an assertion of something that actually happened.

There has, however, always been a tension between what is now and what is to come. On the one hand, there is emphasis on the importance of one's actions in the present, and on the other hand, there is anticipation of some momentous future action of God in the lives of men and women. The Old Testament orientation to the future is subtle and complex and seems to develop in relation to the circumstances of the people. In the early days of the nation, Amos speaks of the day of the Lord that is to come. Later, Jeremiah warns of a future day of judgment. An idealistic outlook develops during the exile, recorded by Second Isaiah. After the exile, the future is pushed farther and farther away, and its manifestation includes supernatural embellishments. Not only does the notion of salvation then become increasingly eschatological (future-oriented), but it also gathers apocalyptic (mysterious, sudden, and dreadful) features. In later Judaism it was even thought that salvation could be earned by following certain formulas, rituals, and patterns of behavior. This behavior essentially overlooked the needs and struggles in the daily lives of the people and, instead, doggedly adhered to actions sanctioned by the legal code. It is when the people relate salvation exclusively to the future, and divorce it from the present, that they become disoriented and provoke the challenge of the prophets, and later of Jesus and Paul.

The idea of future salvation must never be seen as totally new and divorced from the present. Salvation that is to come will be consistent with, and developed from, the salvation that has already been realized. Trust is to be placed in the future because we have experienced present salvation. In a sense we find that our own mighty acts in history establish our present salvation, and from this basis we move forward into our future. Yet, as we do, unless we are either blind or insensitive, we recognize that our community, while eschatologically whole, is presently broken. This recognition of the wholeness that is to come is the stuff of suffering, because it shows us the brokenness and incompleteness of what is. Suffering, we have said, is our homing device, and it strikes its target precisely at the point where our own acts of salvation begin. It strikes where relationships of truth, trust, justice, and love are being forged out of the alienation and incompleteness around them.

There are those who, through the eyes of faith, see their personal salvation both now and in the future. Psychologically this can provide a sense of confidence and sureness in their own life. These same people, with the eyes of flesh, see troubled and broken humanity. Psychologically this can evoke a variety of emotional responses, which may include sadness, anger, fear, or guilt; but whatever the emotion, the experience is one of suffering. These two visions are not necessarily in conflict, but rather, they serve to enhance one another. It is difficult to think that people who are truly convinced of their personal salvation would be anything other than passionately involved with the day-to-day history and struggle of their fellow human beings. Knowledge and experience through faith of one's personal salvation does not insulate one from the knowledge and experience of past and present; rather, it draws one headlong into the turmoil of reality. Salvation is found in meeting and confronting this reality. Pretense and illusion are contrary to salvation, and suffering helps assure that one is not falling into them. In this sense it could be said that it is not only by looking at the sarx that we find the doxa, but it is by looking with the sarx that we find the doxa. Our salvation is found with our suffering. By honestly looking with our eyes of flesh stripped of illusion and pretense, we are able to see glory.

Let us now turn to seek further how these two words, "suffering" and "salvation," may be linked together. We will look briefly at the work of some poets, playwrights, and developmental psychologists, and at some biblical passages.

T. S. Eliot, in *Murder in the Cathedral*, accents the painful paradox of having to take action in ambiguity.

> They know and do not know, what it is to act or suffer.
> They know and do not know, that acting is suffering.[19]

Proust assures us that something positive can be found in reality, no matter how broken it is: "The most terrible reality brings us, with our suffering, the joy of a great discovery."[20] Emily Dickinson suggests that moments of honest pleasure seem to exact a price.

> For each ecstatic instant
> We must an anguish pay

> In keen and quivering ratio
> To the ecstasy.[21]

Keats devotes an entire poem to his struggle with Melancholy. Milton, in his dyad *L'Allegro* and *Il Penseroso,* points to the tension between joy and sorrow, action and thought, as necessary to creation and fulfillment in life.

Needless to say, there are numerous further examples from literature that could be cited which relate suffering to human progress. The notion of suffering moved into political influence with Mahatma Gandhi's explanation of his revolutionary doctrine of nonviolence. Gandhi writes: "For what appears truth to the one may appear to be error to the other. And patience means self-suffering. So the doctrine came to mean vindication of truth, not by infliction of suffering on the opponent, but on one's self."[22]

One of the great pursuits of the behavioral scientist has been to learn how the mind develops from infancy to maturity. Let us look briefly at how two great students and discoverers of the mind, Sigmund Freud and Melanie Klein, help us in our discussion.

Sigmund Freud tells us of the importance of the ego gaining mastery over the id. The id operates under what is referred to as primary-process thinking. The two characteristics of primary-process thinking are the tendency to immediate gratification and the ease by which emotional energy can be shifted from its original object or method of discharge to another object or method of discharge, in the event that the original object or method is blocked. The ego operates under secondary-process thinking, which we could speak of as adult or mature thinking. Adult and mature thinking is rational and logical. It allows for consideration and planning; it is the fabric of civilized and cooperative relationships. Life lived with only primary-process thinking would be chaotic and nonsensical; actions would be taken to assure immediate gratification of our own need without consideration of the consequences. The development of secondary-process thinking comes at the price of enduring the experience of not having one's needs immediately gratified. No satisfactory word was found to explain true feeling of this experience. The German word that Freud used to express the opposite of pleasure is, in English, "unlust," which has often been translated "pain."[23] In order to avoid the misleading connotation of pain, some more recent translators use the clumsy but less ambiguous word "unpleasure." It is interesting how close this comes to the notion of suffering in the way it is being used in our discussion. Unpleasure becomes a component in the development of mature thought and action.

The mature person gradually learns to delay immediate gratification, to tolerate frustration, and so to become civilized. The propensity to violence today leads one to wonder whether or not our culture is too much governed by the need for immediate gratification. However, growth to maturity requires the realization that much of what one wants now, and may even think is deserved now, cannot be attained now. This realization is learned through suffering.

Another psychoanalyst, Melanie Klein, described infants as living in a world of opposites, a world where things are both good and bad. Infants experience themselves either as comfortable or in pain, hungry or satisfied. She pictures them as living in a simplistic world of good and bad, a world for which she uses the image of the good breast and the bad breast. For infants the good breast is the breast that feeds them and the bad breast is that which leaves them hungry. In this simple world there are two unreconcilable opposites, those things which provide and help and those which withhold and punish. She refers to this stage of development as the paranoid stage. As the children mature, they pass through another stage in which it is recognized that the good things are not perfect and the bad things are not horrible. The idealized good breast is no longer so perfect but is also the same one that sometimes does not feed. She refers to this stage as the depressive stage. Once again we are given the message that growth into reality is accompanied by some discomfort. The paranoid stage lends itself to polarization. The depressive stage leads to the acceptance of ambiguity.

There are people who lack the capacity to sustain any mental discomfort or suffering, and when they experience any threat or are faced with more than minimal frustration or inconvenience, they become angry. There seems, for them, to be no solution to painful experience. When they were children, their natural response to pain, whether tears or problem-solving behavior, was probably met by parental anger, neglect, or confusion, which only led to more pain. In such an environment the child is unable to learn and progress through pain, and learns to respond to pain by primitive anger or withdrawal. In order to develop the capacity to suffer, it appears that a person must be able to integrate mental pain and discomfort into the memory and experience. It seems necessary to have experienced solutions to painful problems in the past and to have gained the knowledge that relief from pain is often possible. The solution for children is found mainly through parents and community. Where their parents and community are neglectful and unpredictable, the children will tend to develop mental disturbances or harden into a position of relative inability to suffer. They will likely lack empathy and will feel sad only when they do not get their own way.

Such was the case of a fourteen-and-a-half-year-old who had become increasingly truant, was moving with a delinquent group, and was smoking pot on a regular basis. He described how he and his friends enjoyed vandalizing, removing street signs, and breaking windows. When asked how he felt when he did these things, he replied, "I feel good, it makes me laugh." When asked about his future, he said that he wanted a job and his own apartment so that he could do what he wanted and not get pushed around. He went on: "I'm just waiting for something to happen. It is going to be bad; I know that. I tell lies at home and at school. I'm scared I'm going to get busted; I'm toking a lot."

The awareness of his situation in life only moved him to petulance and fatalism; he lacked the capacity to suffer and so was unable to deal creatively with his life.

His story can be contrasted to that of a sixteen-year-old girl who was hospitalized with severe asthma. She had not had asthma since her family had immigrated to Canada eight years previously. Shortly before this renewed attack her father died. Her mother was also sick, and this girl, the youngest of the family and her father's favorite, was determined to be helpful to the rest of the family. She refused to accept the fact that she too had needs for love and comfort. Her asthma allowed her to be taken care of without having to admit these needs. She was helped to see and accept how everyone has such needs, and was also able to accept that she too had these needs. The way was opened for her to begin to mourn, and her asthma improved. She was able to allow herself to feel mental discomfort, and so she was able to move forward into her own history.

At the individual level the ability to suffer is a mark of personal growth and maturity. It would also seem to be an important ability at the social and interpersonal level. A strong force to unity is a common adversary. To a married couple this adversary may be the illness of a child or the struggle to save money for some common goal. Friendships are often built in a common endeavor to overcome some problem. During such activity, people work toward a goal not yet realized, and while they work, they put aside immediate gratification for the sake of a greater good. During this time they are nourished by their relationships, and at the same time, they are building their relationships—of such is salvation!

One might well monitor the health of a community and nation by measuring its capacity to suffer. Here again one is not measuring masochism; one is not monitoring pain for the sake of pain. What is being measured is the ability honestly to accept the reality of existence. One is reminded of the quality of endurance in the British throughout the dark years of the war, or of the spirit in the people of Israel during the Babylonian captivity. This may be contrasted to the picture of a nation living beyond its means, wasting its resources, and holding up lotteries as the painless means to an empty salvation—a nation that seems to show little capacity to suffer.

Let us turn and look at a group of important passages from the Bible that relate suffering and salvation. These passages are those that set forth the mysterious and mighty figure of the suffering servant. The four passages, often referred to as the servant songs, are all found in the book of the prophet Isaiah and are generally accepted to be Isa. 42:1–4; 49:1–6; 50:4–9; 52:13; 53:12. The ser-

vant is identified as God's chosen one who will
make justice shine on the nations.

> Here is my servant, whom I uphold,
> my chosen one in whom I delight,
> I have bestowed my spirit upon him,
> and he will make justice shine on the nations.
>
> (Isa. 42:1, NEB)

The servant announces his mission; he is Israel.

> He said to me, "You are my servant,
> Israel through whom I shall win glory";
> so I rose to honour in the Lord's sight
> and my God became my strength.
>
> (Isa. 49:3, NEB)

Even though he must suffer violence and igno-
miny, he is confident of his divine vindicator.

> I did not hide my face from spitting and insult;
> but the Lord God stands by to help me;
> therefore no insult can wound me.
> I have set my face like flint,
> for I know that I shall not be put to shame,
> because one who will clear my name is at my side.
>
> (Isa. 50:6–8, NEB)

The servant was disfigured and despised, and people thought that he was stricken by God; but they
saw that it was for their sin and not his own that
the servant died.

> He was despised, he shrank from the sight of men,
> tormented and humbled by suffering;

we despised him, we held him of no account,
a thing from which men turn away their eyes. . . .
But he was pierced for our transgressions,
tortured for our iniquities;
the chastisement he bore is health for us
and by his scourging we are healed.

(Isa. 53:3–5, NEB)

He is a figure who brings salvation to the people.

There are several points of contact between the servant songs and our previous discussion. It is fascinating to consider that these passages were written at a time when psychological and sociological frames of reference, as we have them today, were nonexistent. The scholars of those days, when considering the nature of humankind and the historical situation, used the language of folklore, poetry, and myth available to them. The transactions and tensions between individuals and groups were known and experienced, but there was no technical language to explain them. This, of course, did not mean that their thought patterns were primitive and naive, only that they were different from ours. These early scholars would probably puzzle over the importance we give to the Apollonian-Dionysian controversy (logical thought versus feeling and intuition) or find our bent to uncover scientific fact restrictive to our understanding.

We, however, like them, are locked into the thought patterns of our day. Today we identify both the individual and the group as important in the working out of salvation. Salvation then, in contemporary language, emerges at the individual or psychological level as well as the group or sociological level. This harmonizes with the Old Testament picture of the servant. The problem has always been to decide whether he is a single or corporate individual. Is he one person, or is he the community? It is argued by some that the author intended the servant to be seen as both, in order to stress the important truth that, at the historical level, salvation is achieved in the work of the individual and the group.

A further consideration—the common Christian understanding that the suffering servant is predictive of Jesus should not prevent its application to others. Jesus is said to identify himself with the servant, but this in no sense limits the image to Jesus alone. The wisdom of the prophet has captured a truth that speaks to all humanity. The servant songs hold an eternal truth with which all men and women may identify, and it was an image that Jesus grasped. McClendon talks of the central importance for Dag Hammarskjöld and Martin Luther King of certain momentous images. In the same way, the image of the suffering servant was a momentous one for Jesus and was central in the understanding of his ministry. If such be the case, it follows that the image of the suffering servant should not be absent from the self-identity of those who presume to follow him.

In an attempt to summarize all of what we have been saying in these first four chapters, I am setting forth yet one more image—that of the healer.

The ministry of healing has to do with more than the healing of bodies; it has to do with the healing of lives. Where understanding replaces confusion, where recognition replaces strangeness, where relationship replaces alienation—there is healing. Where there is an experience of healing, there is an experience of salvation.

When we are involved in a healing experience, whether as psychotherapist, pastoral counselor, friend, confessor, or teacher, we are involved in an experience of suffering as well as salvation. There is suffering in hearing the story of brokenness, and there is salvation in healing. There is salvation shared by the person who came to be healed and the person who was privileged to be in the role of healer. At the moment of healing, not one is healed, but all are healed. At the moment of healing all creation moves closer to being whole and complete. We who would heal may do well to remember our own brokenness and be awake to the salvation we receive when those in our care find the courage to take up and affirm the reality that is their lives.

5.
Religion and Mental Health

Religion can both foster and hinder mental health. Those who have a firm religious belief may have no difficulty accepting the notion that religion can promote mental health. What the religious person often forgets, however, is that religion can also hinder mental health. The fact is that religion is a powerful instrument in human affairs and, like power itself, can be either creative or destructive, depending on how it is used.

The word "religion" conjures up many images in people's minds. On the one hand, the images may be those of the Crusades, the Inquisition, holy war, and Jonestown. These are real events in religious history, and when people who only have images such as these in their minds avoid any involvement with religion, it shows good mental health.

On the other hand, religion can be thought of as the foundation for personal wholeness and integrity, as exemplified in the lives of Martin Luther King, Dag Hammarskjöld, Jean Vanier, Mother

Theresa, and countless others who, professing religious belief, live or have lived lives of rich encounter and creativity. If religion is thought of in these terms, then people may be more open to religion.

From the perspective of mental health, religion can be placed in two opposing categories. It can be thought of as an illusion to protect people from recognizing their powerlessness, finitude, and inevitable death, or as the basis for personal integration and orientation in life. In psychological and psychiatric circles, these opposing views are the basis for much of the conflict about religion.

From the practical point of view, religion's influence on mental health can be appraised in the same way as any other influence on people. The chief concern would be to establish whether those who exercise religious influence relate to people primarily as unique individuals who have personal sovereignty, or whether they relate to people primarily as objects for indoctrination and membership into some ideological movement or religious group. The question is whether the main concern is to develop a relationship of mutuality and openness, or to use the other person for personal aggrandizement, prestige, or reassurance.

In this respect, religion is no different from any other influence; once people as persons become secondary to people as objects, institutional disorientation has set in. For example, the orientation of mental health professionals is primarily on improving the mental health of those in their care, and when such professionals begin to see people

primarily as subjects for research or clients to enhance the clinic's reputation, their capacity to promote healing is in jeopardy—they have become
disoriented. The same is true for religious leaders
who are concerned with relationships of meaning
and purpose; when they begin to see people primarily as objects for conversion or indoctrination,
they too have become disoriented. Religious leaders and mental health professionals serve people
best when they start by listening to the people
they purport to serve. The foundation for the mutual support and alliance of religion and mental health is in the common base of concern for
others.

Religion can be seen as that quality in people
which questions the meaning of life. To put it another way, the religious journey begins when one
asks the meaning of all the other journeys of life,
whether the journeys be into action, into thought,
or into relationship. One does not have to belong
to any formal religious organization or church
group to ask such a question, yet there is little
doubt that when one asks such a question one is
thinking religiously.

This question nourishes and enhances mental
health, because it serves as a corrective to feelings
of meaninglessness, which can be so devastating.
Indeed, if one asks what the meaning of life is, one
has already opened the door to the possibility that
life holds meaning. If life does have meaning and
purpose, then it is not absurd, empty, or ephemeral, but real and eventful. History therefore has a

special significance, and not only the history in the history books but the history of each person. This assertion challenges the empty notion that life is primarily experienced for its own sake. People all too often overlook their uniqueness and how it can contribute to the mosaic of community life, and they turn from attempting to express their uniqueness to simply experiencing life. When untempered by honest questioning, their search for more and more experience leads to a life of increasing loneliness and dissatisfaction. Inherent in religious thinking is the belief that life holds meaning and purpose. This belief nurtures mental health.

Another important factor in religion which benefits mental health and which is a result of persistent questioning about the meaning of life is that the center of life is not oneself. This can be said in many different ways: "I am not the center of the universe," "Humankind is my kind," or, in formal religious language, for example, "I believe in God." From the mental health perspective it makes little difference what language is used; the important point is that a person who has made religion a part of his or her life is no longer in isolation. He or she has identified something outside the self which is of great value and importance. Such a position promotes mental health in that it helps to free people from the burden of having to be perfect—superpeople. The demands that people make of themselves—to do it all, to make it all better, to completely understand, to make sense of everything, to overcome all obstacles—are ultimately self-defeating. Self-criticism is common in mentally disturbed people. The difficulty in dealing with it is that the roots are found in the person's belief that he or she actually is, or ought to be, a superperson. If such is the case, it is no wonder that people blame their inadequate performance. The distraught parent, the unhappy schoolgirl, and the irritable boss may all be feeling the bite of self-inflicted criticism. Religion can help people by freeing them to realize and accept that they are not the center of the universe; people can then better accept the fact that everything does not depend on them.

The realization that one is not alone opens people to the importance of relationship. A sense of isolation is crippling to mental health, and religion can speak to that isolation in both theoretical and practical terms. From a theological point of view, one can discuss the importance of the relationship between God and humankind, and the importance of the relationship between persons. Such thinking is often expressed practically in humane and ethical behavior of people toward one another. Such thinking also underlies the important premise that the primary reality of life lies in relationships with other people. When this premise is neglected, the way is open to personal loneliness at the individual level, and sociopolitical upheaval at the community level.

When people work at relating to one another through mutual respect rather than through assumption, coercion, or domination, mental health will be furthered. When care is taken to speak the truth and to patiently work out expectations for one another, the relationship will grow in trust. Trust, truth, and clear expectations are the basis of all healthy relationships. When the spouse demands without listening, the marriage will falter; when parents "tell" their children and never listen, the family will be weakened; when the teenager has no empathy with the parents, disagreements will be destructive; when politicians ignore their electorate, a nation will disintegrate.

The importance of relationship in religion is often found within religious communities themselves. The caring and concern that people within religious groups often have for one another can be of great mutual support. But religious groups are open to the influence of individuals who seek a position of dominance at the expense of another's freedom. A person who is seeking a community may well be attracted to a religious group, whether it be cult or church. It is, in fact, a person's longing for community and relationship that makes him or her most vulnerable to the approaches of the more unscrupulous religious groups. The person is longing for relationship, and the cult is looking for membership—it would seem to be a happy combination. But what is really going on is often not relationship but indoctrination, and the person loses his or her individuality and becomes a number. Someone considering joining a religious cult or community should ask himself or herself, "Will this community help me deal more openly with the struggles of life?" If the community presumes to say that life's struggles will be over or that there will be no more suffering or pain or there will be no serious questions left, then that community is selling escapism and is not likely to have a positive effect on a person's mental health. If, however, the community seems willing to look at the ambiguity of life without demanding final answers, and seems willing to work at forming relationships built on mutual respect, such a community may well benefit mental health.

A religious community can nurture mental health when it takes major events in life, such as birth, marriage, and death, or central experiences of life, such as joy, sorrow, elation, or despair, and through understanding, worship, or ritual provides people with the context and support from which they can affirm these events and experiences. Through liturgy and worship the religious community can take tragic, tumultuous, traumatic, triumphant, and even apparently trivial times in human lives and give them a context from which they can be remembered, given meaning, and integrated more fully into the lives of those who have experienced them. Religious worship promotes mental health when it gives back to the worshiper his or her own experiences, now enriched by the sense that they have been accepted.

Acceptance of all one's past is important if a religious conversion is to be beneficial to mental health. If conversion means that one's past is now to be forgotten and that somehow one becomes a brand-new person, free from any connections to the past, then conversion has been detrimental to personal growth. Even if conversion means that people are free from only those things they wish to forget, it is still detrimental. Conversion that is beneficial to mental health is an experience that enables a person to integrate past experience, the good with the bad, into oneself in a way that is enriching.

In a healthy conversion, the past becomes nurturing and not encumbering, and instead of forgetting one's roots, one in compassion accepts them. A person is led not to disown the past self and become someone new, but rather to achieve a deeper and more complete integration of the self that was always there. Religious conversion has been detrimental to mental health when the person becomes more simplistic and less tolerant of the ambiguities of life. It has been beneficial when a person can look at reality from a deeper perspective and is better able to form opinions and make decisions out of the ambiguities in which life is found.

Another way religion can be beneficial to mental health is by protecting people from magic— magical thinking, magical leaders, magical theories, magical solutions. Life is ambiguous, and absolute certitude, security, and perfection are unattainable. It is understandable that people in fear, confusion, uncertainty, and despair would want the easy and permanent relief promoted by our culture. But such relief is an illusion. It would be magic if the government or parents or therapists could really take away our problems. It would be magic if by treatment of the teenager we could overcome the effects of child abuse and neglect. It would be magic if there really was a solution to every problem. In support of such magic is the contemporary conjurers' trick of reducing the ambiguities of life to a "simple clear analysis" and then providing "the answer" to the problems posed.

Psychiatrists and mental health professionals are often confronted by distraught parents who say they have been unsuccessful in finding help for their child and now they really want to get to "the root of the problem." Others may say, "They can put a man on the moon, why can't they make my son stop his angry outbursts?" The answer is that putting a man on the moon may well be easier. There is no one "root" to most human problems. The problems are the result of a complex interaction of biological, sociological, cultural, and psychological factors. To talk as if there really is a "root" to a human problem is illusory and holds out the myth of a "cure." Health is to be found in an honest dealing with all the issues involved and in an acceptance that the wished-for cure exists only in the bottom of the magician's bag of tricks.

Contemporary magicians wear many disguises, and some who are dressed in the clothing of religion promote supernatural solutions to life's difficulties. No matter what the source of illusion, the effect is detrimental to mental health. There are, however, few people who would not be delighted if all their problems could be taken care of painlessly. When religion is operating with integrity, however, it challenges illusions, because the religious position is not embarrassed to say that evil is real. From the perspective of religion, evil must be reckoned with; life will not be made better simply by asking people to be nice to one another. Because evil is real, the ideal is not attainable. The acceptance of evil as real does not push one to a flurry of guilt or to withdrawal in resignation. Instead, it opens one to an acceptance of reality. The health of the individual and the community is fostered when they work with what is available and do not pine for magical solutions.

It is the nonreligious use of the word "hope" that is so misleading. When hope is based on magic, it becomes the energy that keeps people looking for the impossible and the painless solution. The family does not give up hope, and so they go from clinic to clinic. The individual does not give up hope, and so goes through drugs, cults, meditation, and diets. Neither the family nor the individual is willing to persist in dealing with the reality of the situation; hope has become a magical distraction. Hope in the religious sense holds a quite different meaning, because it is based on the assurance that progress comes when people base their action on what is there and not on what they wish was there.

Hope is, after all, the twin, the other side of the coin, the warp to the woof of courage. Courage and hope are inseparable. Where we find one, we will find the other; where one is absent, so is the other. The gift of courage becomes the gift of hope. When we have courage, we can hope; in the absence of courage there is hopelessness. When we despair of finding a solution, it is to magic and to wishful thinking that we appeal, not to hope. Hope is based on courage, and courage is found in facing what is there, not in turning from it. Hope tells us that any circumstance, no matter how dreadful, will have healing somewhere when it is met with honesty.

A fifty-five-year-old man came all the way to the big city from his home in the bush; he had flagged down the train at the whistle-stop. He came because his doctor had told him that the specialists in the city would help him. In his arms he carried the X-rays his doctor had given him. At the hospital, the specialist put the X-rays into the viewer and then said to him: "What are you doing here? There is nothing we can do. Go back home and make out your will." The man's lungs were full of cancer. He could see no hope. In spite of his tears and shock, he managed to get into a conversation with a nurse. It lasted several hours and covered many parts of his life, but through it all the word "hope" kept reappearing. After spending that night in the hospital, in the morning the man thanked the nurse and said that he now knew what hope meant. He told her that he intended to go home and tell his wife everything, even though it would be difficult for her. He also wanted to go hunting at least one more time with his friends and to see as much of the spring as possible. And he told the nurse that for the last two months he had been unable to sleep well, but that this past night he had slept peacefully.

This story shows that hope can never be found in magic, that it is to be found in life itself. Hope serves mental health when it is used in a religious sense, that is, when it is based on the assurance that when issues are faced honestly and with courage some healing will take place. Out of brokenness some union will emerge, out of strangeness some recognition, out of confusion some clarity.

Religion can help people to find a deeper meaning in life, to grow into relationships of deeper commitment, and to find their hope by facing reality, not in magic. Because religion can open men and women to the gift of courage, it has profound consequences for mental health and for the shape of life itself.

Notes

1. The literature in the area of psychiatry and religion is extensive, and to give only a few examples is an arbitrary procedure. The following is a diverse sampling that might be of interest:

Gordon W. Allport, *The Individual and His Religion: A Psychological Interpretation* (London: Constable & Co., 1951). This famous author discusses the ways in which religion develops from youth to adolescence and through into maturity.

Malcolm Jeeves, *Psychology and Christianity: The View Both Ways* (Inter-Varsity Press, 1976). An elementary but clear exposition of the essential issues between psychology and Christianity. It provides useful references.

H. Newton Malony (ed.), *Current Perspectives in the Psychology of Religion* (Wm. B. Eerdmans Publishing Co., 1977). A collection of fifteen papers, all written within the past fifteen years, showing the broad range of contemporary viewpoints.

Rollo May, *Love and Will* (Dell Publishing Co.,

1973). This well-known author and therapist examines these moral issues from the psychological point of view.

Karl Menninger, *Whatever Became of Sin?* (Bantam Books, 1978). This famous psychiatrist looks at the tendency of contemporary analysis and classification to explain sin away.

Michael Novak, *Ascent of the Mountain, Flight of the Dove* (Harper & Row, 1971). A sensitive and searching look into the impact of religion at the very depth of human life.

B. F. Skinner, *Beyond Freedom and Dignity* (Bantam Books, 1972). In contradiction to the Christian view of humanity, this book reduces human behavior to the operation of simple cause and effect.

Other publications will be referred to throughout the book.

2. C. J. Jung, *Collected Works,* Vol. II (Princeton University Press, 1958), p. 168.

3. Aleksandr Solzhenitsyn, *The Gulag Archipelago, Two* (Harper & Row, 1975), p. 615.

4. Paul Ricoeur, *The Symbolism of Evil* (Beacon Press, 1969).

5. Paul Tillich, *The Courage to Be* (Yale University Press, 1961).

6. Sam Keen, "The Herosis of Everyday Life: A Conversation with Ernest Becker," *Psychology Today,* Vol. 7, No. 11 (April 1974), p. 80.

7. Tillich, *The Courage to Be,* p. 77.

8. Hans Küng, *On Being a Christian* (Glasgow: William Collins & Co., 1978), p. 516.

9. Erik H. Erikson, *Identity and the Life Cycle,* Psy-

chological Issues Monograph, Vol. 1, No. 1 (1959), p. 63.

10. C. G. Jung (ed.), *Man and His Symbols* (Double-day & Co., 1964).

11. Rollo May, "Symbols for Our Future," a recorded address.

12. Viktor E. Frankl, *Man's Search for Meaning* (Washington Square Press, 1963), p. 131.

13. James W. McClendon, Jr., *Biography as Theology* (Abingdon Press, 1974).

14. Herbert O'Driscoll, an address given at 53d Weekend, London, Ontario, May 1976, and recorded by the Diocese of Huron.

15. Rudolf Bultmann, *The Gospel of John* (Oxford: Basil Blackwell, Publisher, 1971; Philadelphia: Westminster Press, 1971), p. 63.

16. From a sermon by the Rev. David Ward, at St. Paul's Memorial Church, Charlottesville, Virginia, Sunday, March 28, 1976.

17. St. Augustine, *Confessions* (Penguin Books, 1979), p. 21.

18. Alan Richardson, "Salvation," *Interpreter's Dictionary of the Bible* (Abingdon Press, 1962), pp. 168–181.

19. T. S. Eliot, *Murder in the Cathedral* (London: Faber & Faber, 1950), p. 21.

20. Marcel Proust, *Remembrance of Things Past. Cities of the Plain,* Pt. II (Random House, 1934).

21. Emily Dickinson, *Complete Poems,* ed. by Thomas H. Johnson (Little, Brown & Co., 1960).

22. Mahatma Gandhi, *Defense Against Charge of Sedition,* March 23, 1922.

23. Charles Brenner, *An Elementary Textbook of Psychoanalysis* (Doubleday & Co., 1957), pp. 72ff.